HCG Approved Summer Spritzers: You Can Still Enjoy Delicious Alcoholic Beverages on the HCG Diet

Disclaimer and Terms of Use: Effort has been made to ensure that the information in this book is accurate and complete, however, the author and the publisher do not warrant the accuracy of the information, text and graphics contained within the book due to the rapidly changing nature of science, research, known and unknown facts and Internet. The Author and the publisher do not hold any responsibility for errors, omissions or contrary interpretation of the subject matter herein. This book is presented solely for motivational and informational purposes only.

Table of Contents

Mint Sauce (yes, a drink)

Ingredients:

- 2 mint sprigs
- 4 - 8 drops Stevia
- ice
- 2 oz. bourbon

Directions:

I. Add everything together in a glass, sometimes adding ice first is best
II. Fill the glass ¾ full
III. Enjoy without the calorie guilt!

Lonkero

Ingredients:
- 1 T gin
- 3 T grapefruit Juice
- ½ tsp. lemon juice
- 6 drops Stevia
- 1 C sparkling water

Directions:

I. Add everything together in a glass, sometimes adding ice first is best
II. Fill the glass ¾ full
III. Enjoy without the calorie guilt!

Ingredients:

- 1 oz. Vodka
- 1 oz. lemon juice
- 6 drops Stevia
- 4 oz. sparking water

Directions:

I.   Add everything together in a glass, sometimes adding ice first is best
II.   Fill the glass ¾ full
III. Enjoy without the calorie guilt!

Ravenous Raspberry

Ingredients:
- 1 ½ oz. light rum
- 2 oz. crushed raspberries
- 16 drops Stevia
- 1 t lime juice
- ¾ C water

Directions:

I.   Add everything together in a glass, sometimes adding ice first is best

II. Fill the glass ¾ full

III. Enjoy without the calorie guilt!

Cherry Bomb

Ingredients:

- 2 tsp. cherry syrup
- 16 drops Stevia
- 2 oz. light rum
- ¼ C Crushed ice

Directions:

I. Add everything together in a glass, sometimes adding ice first is best
II. Fill the glass ¾ full
III. Enjoy without the calorie guilt!

Savory Citrus

Ingredients:
- 1 tsp. lemon juice
- 1 tsp. grated lime peel
- 1 tsp. orange peel
- 16 drops Stevia

Directions:

I. Add everything together in a glass, sometimes adding ice first is best
II. Fill the glass ¾ full
III. Enjoy without the calorie guilt!

Ingredients:
- 1 C crushed ice
- 1 oz. vodka
- 1 oz. heavy cream
- 1 tsp. coffee granules
- 12 Stevia drops

Directions:

I.   Add everything together in a glass, sometimes adding ice first is best

II.   Fill the glass ¾ full

III.   Enjoy without the calorie guilt!

Sour Apple

Ingredients:
- 2 tsp. cherry Stevia
- 1 ¼ C pressed apple juice
- 4 C water

Directions:

I. Add everything together in a glass, sometimes adding ice first is best

II. Fill the glass ¾ full

III. Enjoy without the calorie guilt!

Cherry Cinnamon

Ingredients:
- 2 oz. heavy cream
- 1 tsp. cherry flavor
- 8 - 10 drops Stevia
- ground cinnamon

Directions:

I. Add everything into your blender or food processor and blend until smooth
II. Pour into a tall glass and enjoy

Silver Fizz

Ingredients:
- 2 oz. dry gin
- 1 egg white
- ½ T Stevia
- ½ oz. lemon juice
- 2 oz. soda water

Directions:

I.   Add everything together in a glass, sometimes adding ice first is best

II.   Fill the glass ¾ full

III.   Enjoy without the calorie guilt!

Lady Liberty

Ingredients:
- 2 oz. syrup
- rosemary spring
- 4 oz. bourbon
- 2 oz. lemon juice
- 1 T raw syrup
- 1 T orange juice
- 2 T orange marmalade
- 1 egg white

Directions:

I. Boil the syrup and rosemary and let cool
II. Throw away your rosemary and pour everything into shaker with the bourbon
III. Add everything else into glass
IV. Add ice

Summer Spritzer

Ingredients:
- 3 oz. Prosecco
- 1 ½ oz. Aperol
- 1 ½ oz. soda water

Directions:

Combine everything together and garnish with fruit wedge

Antebellum Julep

Ingredients:
- 2 T Stevia
- mint leaves
- 2 T Julep
- 2 oz. Cognac

Directions:

I.   Stir Stevia add water and Julep until sugar dissolves
II.   Add mint leaves
III.   Add Cognac and ice

Heat Snapper

Ingredients:
- 2 oz. Cognac
- ½ oz. lemon juice
- 1 tsp. crème de farmhouse
- 1 tsp. raw honey
- ½ orange slice to taste

Directions:

Add everything to shaker and enjoy

Apple Spray

Ingredients:
- 1 ½ T fennel seeds
- 1 C Stevia
- 1 C water
- ¼ C apple juice
- 1 T lemon juice
- 1 ¼ C sparkling water
- apple, sliced

Directions:

I. Start with your syrup
II. Grind the fennel and add remaining ingredients and set over heat
III. Bring to a boil and remove from heat
IV. Strain and let sit for 30 minutes
V. Make the spritzer, add everything to gather, stirring well
VI. Serve

White Punch, With a Bite

Ingredients:
- 2 oz. white whiskey
- 2 oz. pineapple juice
- 1 oz. lime juice
- 1 oz. pineapple syrup

Directions:

I.   Mix everything together and chill, add to shaker
II.   Shake, pour and serve

Sour Slushy

Ingredients:
- 2 C water
- 1 1/3 C Stevia
- 1 C lime juice
- 1/2 C lemon juice
- 1/2 C Yuzu juice
- 1/3 C Pisco

Directions:

I.   Make the syrup by bringing water and Stevia to a boil, stir until it dissolves
II.   Refrigerate and add in remaining ingredients
III.   Wait for it to freeze and blend
IV.   Serve

Black Tea

Ingredients:
- 6 oz. fruit flavored iced tea
- 1 ½ oz. gin
- white peach, sliced

Directions:

I.   Add everything together in a glass and serve cold
II.   Top with seltzer

Goblin Gin

Ingredients:
- 2 oz. Spanish banjo
- 1 1/2 oz. rum
- 3/4 oz. lime juice
- 3/4 C ice
- 2 tsp. grapefruit juice
- 1 tsp. cinnamon syrup
- 1 tsp. Grenadine
- 1/8 tsp. period
- 1 mint sprig

Directions:

I.   Add everything together in a bowl without the mint
II.   Blend on high
III.   Pour into glass and garnish with the mint sprig

Pink Flamingo

Ingredients:
- 2 oz. white rum
- ¾ oz. lime juice
- 3 oz. grapefruit soda
- 1 lime slice to garnish

Directions:

I.   Add everything into your shaker
II.   Shake well and serve
III.   Add lime wedge to garnish

Raspberry Punch

Ingredients:
- 3 oz. dry gin
- 1 oz. syrup
- 1 oz. lemon juice
- 6 raspberries
- soda water

Directions:

I.   Add everything to martini shaker (but your soda water), shake and pour into glass

II. Top off with soda water

The Smash

Ingredients:
- 3 lemon wedges
- 3 mint leaves
- 1 oz. rhubarb syrup
- 1 ½ oz. bourbon
- 1 ½ strawberries, stemmed

Directions:

I.   Mix everything and add syrup to the bottom of your glass
II.   Add bourbon and the ice
III.   Serve cold

Herb Spritzer

Ingredients:
- 2 ½ oz. fruitable jasmine
- 8 oz. seltzer
- 8 - 10 Stevia drops
- 1 lemon, wedged

Directions:

I.   Fill a mason jar and add first 3 ingredients, add lid and shake
II.   Add remaining ingredients and stir

Lemon Fizz

Ingredients:
- 1 C Stevia
- 1 C water
- 1 lavender tea bag
- 2 oz. gin
- 1 ½ oz. lavender syrup
- ¾ oz. lemon juice
- club soda

Directions:

I.   Add lavender tea bag in water and bring to a boil
II.   Remove from heat and steep
III.   Add in remaining ingredients

Green Cooler

Ingredients:
- 1 cucumber, diced
- 1/8 tsp. thyme leaves
- 1 /12 oz. Vodka
- 1/2 oz. syrup

Directions:

I.   Add everything to a shaker and shake
II.   Add ingredients as needed
III.   Serve cold

www.ingramcontent.com/pod-product-compliance
Lightning Source LLC
Chambersburg PA
CBHW070941290526
45795CB00003B/1101